Also by Dr. Stenbeck

Available from the usual on-line source

Books
Healing Yourself -- The Holistic Approach
    [An introduction to Holistic Self-healing.]

Heal Yourself Right Now!
    [The Seven Priority Organ Levels for
    effective Nutritional/Holistic Treatment of
    all organs.]

The 22 Unique Body Types
    (for Health and Weight Loss)

Q & A to Identify Your Body Type (Booklet)
    [Individual Type booklets are also available

Booklets
(Step-by-step instructions on healing yourself)

    #1 Start Healing with Positive Thinking
    #2 Mastering Positive Feelings for Health!
    #3 Spiritual Balance and Your Healing

The Isogenic Body Type

*Representing one of the 22 Body
Types first described by Victor
Rocine around 1900*

The
Phillip S .Hoffman,
Oprah Winfrey
Celebrity Body Type

For Kaye,
there at the beginning with Doc Severn,
and for Liberty,
continuing the holistic healing journey...

Disclaimer

The information in this book is for educational purposes only and is not a substitute for medication, diets, or other medical care. The diets do not treat diseases or medical conditions, and are an adjunct to your orthodox health care.

The author and publisher accept no responsibility for any misuse of the information within. If you have any physical problem, food allergy, emotional disorder, or disease, common sense dictates that you consult with a physician before changing your diet, taking nutritional supplements, or following the advice given here.

———

About the Author

Educated in New Zealand and in the U.S.A., Dr. Stenbeck attained B.Sc. (NZ), M.S., and D.C. degrees. His holistic healing methods have been profiled in magazines (Esquire, McLean's, Playgirl, the Atlanta Constitution), and on TV in the USA and in Canada. He was the main contributor to the Warner Book, _The Eye/Body Connection_ by Jessica Maxwell that focused on the holistic healing relationships between the iris structure and organ genetics.

In the 1970-80's he was elected Fellow, Royal Society of Health, London; Fellow, American Association of Chemists; Member, American Association of Clinical Chemists; and Affiliate, Royal Society of Medicine, London. He studied naturopathy and Body Types with Dr. Bernard Jensen and Dr. Clifford Severn, and has practiced in medical partnerships where patients received the joint benefits of medical and holistic healing.

He is a member of Self-Realization Fellowship. To receive advice on any health issue from a holistic viewpoint, or to receive help with your body type, see his web site: *DrStenbeck.net*

———

Contents

* * *

The Isogenic Body Type and Food Guide   *1*

* * *

The 22 Body Types:
Celebrity Examples

This Booklet contains the Isogenic type. See <u>*The 22 Unique Body Types*</u> *for all type descript-ions.]*

Thin Types

Atrophic   *Woody Allen / Audrey Hepburn*
             Stan Laurel / Calista Flockheart

Exesthesic   *Cher / Sarah Jessica Parker*
             (Female type only)

Marasmic   *President Obama / Princess Diana*
             James Stewart / Kate Blanchard

Neurogenic   *J.K. Simmons / Joan Rivers*
             Jon Cryer / Marin Hinle

Pathoferic   *(No celebrity males)*
             Blythe Danner / Gwyneth Paltrow

Sillevitic   *David Bowie / Shirley MacLaine*
             Rod Stewart / Carol Channing

Muscle Types

Calciferic   *Michael Jordan / Angelica Huston*
                 Abraham Lincoln / Grace Jones

Carbogenic   *George Clooney / Lady Gaga*
                 Pres. G. Bush, Jr. / Meg Ryan

Desmogenic   *Marlon Brando / Loni Anderson*
                 Daniel Craig / Tina Turner

Eldic   *Ross Perot / Hillary Clinton*
                 Peter Falk / Sigourney Weaver

Medeic   *Gary Oldman / Madonna*
                 John Hurt / Marlene Deitrich

Myogenic   *Pres. Bill Clinton / Sharon Stone*
                 Pres. John Kennedy / Julia Roberts

Nervimotive   *Frank Sinatra / Elizabeth Taylor*
                 Mark Wahlberg / Natalie Wood

Nitropheric   *Ben Affleck / Ava Gardner*
                 Kirk Douglas / Kate Winslet

Pallinomic   *Pres. Donald Trump /*
                 Attorney General Janet Reno
                 Bill O'Reilly (Fox) / Jane Russell

Fat Types

Barotic

Robin Williams / 'Mrs.Doubtfire'
Elton John / William Conrad

Carboferic

Bill Murray / Roseanne
Billy Gardell / Melissa McCarthy

Hydripheric

John Goodman / Shelly Winters
Wayne Knight / Jennifer Holliday

Isogenic

Einstein / Oprah Winfrey
Phillip S .Hoffman / Queen Victoria

Lipopheric

Rush Limbaugh / Rosie O'Donnell
Chris Christie / Camryn Manheim

Oxypheric

Winston Churchill / Orsen Welles
Ella Fitzgerald / Gerry Spence

Pargenic

Burt Reynolds / Katey Segal
Ron Perlman / Kirstey Alley

<u>*Succinct Quote on Human Types*</u>

From Victor Rocine, who first described discrete body types around 1900.

"A type is an order of people that differentiates and distinguishes itself by a general and similar form, brain-formation, chemistry, structure, build, immunity, tendencies, predisposition, resemblance, skin-pigment, and type characteristics based on observation and analogy.

"Or, in other words, people of a given type are similar physically and like-minded as if they were brothers and sisters—that is what type means.

"Everything in nature is made according to plan. Man only discovers that plan and gives it a name. The zoologist has not made the animals—he has only described the plan adopted by the wonderful Creator, and named the classes, sub-classes, etc.

"How important type research will be to humanity, time alone will make known."

———

Prologue

The esteemed scientist J. J. Berzelius, discoverer of several chemical elements, inspired Victor Rocine to research body types and to investigate the correlation between types and their diseases. Around 1890-1910, Rocine privately published his original findings on the mineral basis of different body types, and this present book exists because of his brilliant insights.

For many years, I studied with Dr. Clifford Severn who had been a personal student of Victor Rocine on body types, naturopathy, herbology, iris analysis, diet, and nutritional healing methods. He had a successful career as a lecturer and healer, and was one of those rare athletes with complete muscle control over his body. I saw him under a spotlight at 85 years of age, contracting and rippling every individual muscle in his perfectly developed body. Field-Marshal Jan Smuts, the WWII South African Prime Minister, devoted a full chapter of his autobiography to how Severn's healing methods had saved his life. In the 1950's, *Life* magazine did a four-page spread on Severn and his family. Fame he had.

Another Rocine student I studied with, Dr. Bernard Jensen wrote of Rocine's body type research and nutritional methods in his privately published, *The Chemistry of Man*.

This book is deeply rooted in Rocine's original work, and with that of Herbert Shelton, M.D., Ph.D. (at Harvard University in the 1930's). I integrated their research with newer dietary and nervous system data along with celebrity examples of each type, hopefully, making this material easier to digest and more entertaining for the reader.

Gayelord Hauser, another Rocine student I knew, was a celebrated health book author. He wrote a popular book on Rocine's types in the 1940's, *Types and Temperaments;* reputedly, he also introduced yogurt to the western world.

This book exists because of Rocine's creative brilliance and original discoveries in natural healing.

▶ *Rocine: "The soul creates the body type."*

Rocine taught that the soul chooses a body type and brain to live in, thus presenting different experiences and life lessons to master. Why were *you* born the way you are?

That is something to think about, especially if it is true! What would your soul purpose be to live in a particular body type. I provide some thoughts on this issue in each type description and try to assess from my experience with your type the particular lessons of life presented therein.

Rocine was as brilliant in his way as an Abraham Lincoln, Michael Jordan, Michael Phelps, Tony Robbins, or a Daniel Day Lewis—all *calciferic* types—rare, leaders, innovative, brilliant, and highly intelligent in their different fields of endeavor.

Celebrity examples exist for most types, not a duplicate of you, but someone who has your essence in their body-mind individuality. Knowing your type allows you to become a better you!

The celebrity examples provide further help in identifying your body type.

▶ *Rocine's classic findings are the backbone of this book. Integrated with Sheldon's research and with other dietary and food issues including mental, emotional, and spiritual attributes,*

Many people take nutritional supplements and try different diets without a doctor's advice. If this is your choice, use common sense, listen to body responses, and discontinue any allergic reactions to foods or nutritional substances.

———

The Isogenic
Body Type

"*You may also have a physical or psychological feature not representative of your type such as height, weight, appearance, talent, weakness, strength, etc., due to biochemical errors, environmental influences, racial or cultural differences, and congenital or genetic issues. Nevertheless, the type identification of the average person is usually clear.*"

—*Victor Rocine*

Isogenic Type Celebrity Examples

*If you think this is your type, be sure to look at **on-line photographs** of these examples. Look for general similarities to yourself. Note that sub-types cause the differences in appearance between members of the same type. This is a relatively rare type with few celebrity examples, but the following are highly representative.*

———

GENIUS

Albert Einstein
Thomas Edison

POLITICS

Steve Bannon

ACTOR

Phillip Seymour Hoffman

BUSINESS

Andrew Carnegie

TV/FILM

Oprah Winfrey

ARTS

> Maeve Binchy (author)
> Neil de Grosse Tyson (science)
> Toni Morrison (author)

HISTORY (by Rocine)

> Arthur Conan Doyle
> George Eliott
> Queen Victoria (very typical of how the females may look by middle age)

[Note: I personally knew several members of this type who were all quite heavy, all of which contributed to my understanding of the type.

Read through the types, and if still confused see the *Appendix,* for the personal type identification request from my website: *DrStenbeck.net*

———

Isogenic Type Questionnaire

These questions describe the generic type, and not specifically you! If any question ever applied to you, then choose the True answer!

For Question 1 only:

A = True	*B = Maybe*	*C = Untrue*
15 points	*7 points*	*1 point*

1. Physically identify with celebrity example____

Then...

A = True	*B = Maybe*	*C = Untrue*
5 points	*3 points*	*1 point*

---

2. Height is close to:
   Males: 5'7-6'0   Females: 5'5-5'11   ____
3. Usual weight is close to:
   Males: 150-250+ Females: 140-250+   ____
4. Fleshy body, fat or obese; weight
   problems in females from age 25-30;
   in males after age 30-40   ____
5. Muscles compact and strong   ____
6. May be addiction-prone (especially
   males to pot, sex, drugs, or alcohol)   ____
7. Mental work, highly intelligent, intellect ____
8. Positive and optimistic   ____

9. Long body, shorter arms and legs (are taller sitting, shorter on standing) _____
10. Have a loud voice, may be heard across a crowded room _____
11. Benevolent, shy, and kind _____
12. Look peaceful and quiet _____
13. Square, large head, high crown _____
14. While talking, often move head, smile and laugh a lot _____
15. Head average or smaller in males; larger in females _____
16. Fair or brown hair, usually thin, early graying _____
17. Eyebrows typically wide, stiff, bushy _____
18. May be misjudged by lazy posture or a care-free voice _____
19. Long wide face typical; cheekbones, jaws larger and fleshy; cheeks may be sunken with a wide chin _____
20. Wide mouth compared to size of face; upper lip full _____
21. Large, strong teeth; may yellow with aging _____
22. Skin thick; acne, boils history (common in males) _____
23. Nose usually wide and fleshy _____
24. Large chest; small-medium bust; males have minimal chest hair _____
25. Longer from eyes to the mouth (opposite to *hydripheric*) _____
26. Extremities shorter, fatty muscles _____
27. Strong shoulders, wedge-shape to feet _____

28. Hands are short, square, hard, bony _____
29. Have strong will-power, poor memory ____
30. Benevolent, humanitarian; want to
    help the planet _____
31. Highly combative; appear peaceful
    and placid, but are a sleeping storm;
    when aroused, may erupt with fury _____
32. Secretive; need private time alone _____
33. Combative, demanding if provoked _____
34. Deep thinkers, philosophers, think
    and ponder, slow to take action _____
35. May have addictions and cravings _____
36. History of intestine irritation,
    constipation, toxicity, etc. _____
37. Appear laid-back and passive; may be
    aggressive if crossed _____
38. 'Wishy-washy': what is said is not
    necessarily done! _____
39. Are 'self-made': a powerful mind
    and intellect (if not lazy!) _____
40. High sex drive _____
41. Understand principles, natural laws _____
42. Desire to spend time doing nothing,
    procrastinating, plan on relaxing! _____
43. Sensitive; remember hurts _____
44. Are enduring: if maimed in battle
    are never conquered _____
45. Metaphysical, interest in the unknown,
    new age healing _____
46. May have history of lymph congestion,
    boils, colds in childhood _____

47. Formal education is difficult; learn
    slowly and then achieve all goals   _____
48. Great work-ethic; work long hours   _____
49. Strongly desire fame and fortune   _____
50. Vitality and strength when healthy   _____
51. High executive and leadership values   _____
52. Know no failure; keep trying until
    successful   _____
53. History of itching sensations, or pain
    in back, feet, knees, other areas   _____
54. History of pancreas weakness
    (leading to sugar craving, diabetes or
    hypoglycemia)   _____
55. Sports-minded in youth but not
    particularly as adults   _____
56. May talk for hours; are fine teachers   _____

                        _____

▶ *The type questionnaire pinpoints the major features of that type: if the celebrity examples are unhelpful, you may be an unusual variant (in which case ignore the celebrity issue and give yourself 7 points on Question 1).*

Scoring

For question #1:

A response: give 15 points   = _____

B response: give 7 points   = _____

C response: give 1 points   = _____

For questions #2—56:

A response: give 5 points   = _____

B response: give 3 points   = _____

C response: give 1 point   = _____

Total of the above points   = _____

Interpretation

***132—260:* PROBABLY Isogenic type**

59—131:   POSSIBLY Isogenic type

<59:   NOT Isogenic type

The Isogenic Type

Rocine: "Isogenic means even production of brain, fat, and muscle." You utilize more food magnesium, calcium, and carbon than other types leading to brain power and fat development. You are creative, highly intelligent, and a relatively rare body type.

I f female, you may be heavy-set, fat or obese, some from an early age: you rarely learn how to control your fat deposition or find the willpower to help yourself. The males remain lean and muscular looking until age 30-40, after which they may steadily gain weight (if not exercising and eating sensibly. It is difficult to identify your type because you are somewhat uncommon in the United States.

Magnesium and calcium have a stimulating effect on the brain evoking intense thinking, nervousness, and sometimes brilliance.

▶ *Rocine: "You are opposite to the hydripheric in that your lymphatic system is weak, inactive, and vulnerable to disease."*

There are few female celebrities, the brilliant Oprah Winfrey being an excellent example: the world knows of her diet and fat struggles after being a slender beautiful young woman. At the time of this writing her weight is under good control, she is working out, on a diet, etc. However, when and if she stops exercising and dieting she may easily gain weight. Being in the public eye is life saving by providing the motivation she needs to control her weight. The average *isogenic* lady does not have such motivation!

Male examples are scarce, but Phillip Seymour Hoffman, Thomas Edison and Albert Einstein are shining examples. Of course, few of us are that brilliant, but you have a strong creative intelligence!

You may have addictive personality, some males being vulnerable to alcohol, marijuana, or drug addiction.

————

Physical Similarity to Other Types

The fat *carboferic* type (John Goodman, Roseanne Barr) is somewhat similar, but is usually more fatty, approachable, and friendlier.

The *lipopheric* type (Jackie Gleason, Ricki Lake) is usually large, intellectual, and talkative, like the *isogenic*.

The *oxypheric* type (Winston Churchill, Ella Fitzgerald) is naturally expressive and warmly outgoing with a larger forehead and jaw.

The *barotic* type (Robin Williams, "Mrs. Doubtfire") is rotund, sometimes obese, but more reticent, quiet and peaceful.

Younger male *isogenics* may be confused with several of the Muscle types.

Average Height and Weight

The males are generally of medium-height: those I have known were all around 5'7, with taller females.

Males: 5'7-6'0 150-250+
Females: 5'5-5'11 140-250+

▶ *Rocine: "You usually have shorter legs, making you taller on sitting, and shorter on standing." I have seen this feature many times, particularly in males.*

You already know something about this type from their public persona and appearance, whether from seeing them yourself or from the celebrity examples. Blend such insights with the type descriptions and the types of your family and friends to discern their presence in your midst!

Isogenic Type Description

The type description represents how you appear in everyday society. You may have a sub-type that alters parts of this description.

Think of the celebrity examples as you read the descriptions.

The central body is long, large, and strong. You are plain or homely looking, and pregnant with potential for achievement in the creative, inventive, scientific, or artistic fields.

Head — Your head is average-sized (or smaller) compared to the rest of the body; the forehead is square and large compared to the size of the face; there is a high crown.

Hair — The hair has mostly fair or brown colors, with a stiff, straight texture, and is often prematurely gray.

Eyes — Usually your eyes are blue, some brown; the expression is happy and pleasing. The eyebrows are often wide, stiff, and bushy.

Ears — Various ear shapes and positions are common.

Nose —The nose is usually wide and fleshy.

Face — The cheekbones and jaws are large and fleshy. Your cheeks may be sunken, the chin large and wide.

▶ *Rocine: "A wide face is usual, especially long from the eyes to the mouth." (Opposite to the other fat types.) "You tend to move your head, joke and smile a lot while talking."*

Mouth, Lips and Voice — Your mouth tends to be wider than average; the upper lip is thin, the lower lip fuller. Like the *carboferic and neurogenic* types, you may talk for hours; you are fine teachers.

▶ *When excited, your voice is often characteristically louder than normal; you may be heard from far away (and don't realize it).*

Teeth — Large and strong teeth are usual; you have strong calcium metabolism producing healthy long-surviving teeth (which may yellow with age).

Skin — Your skin is thick and strong, white or gray colored.

Neck — A muscular neck is usual.

Muscles — You have moderate strength.

Chest — The chest and central body is large; the bust is medium-sized or larger; the males have minimal chest hair.

Back and Shoulders — A broad, long and strong back is usual; the shoulders are thick, strong, and rounded; the males show a characteristic wedge-shape from the shoulders to the feet.

Hips and Abdomen — Narrow hips and waist typify the male physique in young adults; the females have bony hips with fat accumulation often from a young age, or by their 30's.

Arms and Legs — You have a long body, well-muscled, short, and with heavy extremities (fatty in females). The hands are large, short, square, hard, and bony; the bones are large, and well padded with flesh.

Joints — Your large bones and joints are strong and stiff.

Weight — The females have a very difficult time with weight and may become quite large with a mixture of water and fat clogging the lymphatic system and engorging all tissues. The males lose weight more easily, exercise being a key in both sexes.

———

Isogenic Personality Traits

If you are this type many, but not all, of the following characteristics are present—you may have overcome or moderated the negatives, but recognize that you once had several of them.

You have many of the following positive traits (when healthy):

- Have a great work ethic
- May join unorthodox religions
- You try, try, try again until successful
- Honesty and integrity are important to you
- Are 'self-made': a powerful mind and intellect
- Are attracted to antiquity and old things of value
- Often interested in metaphysics and the unknown
- Are secretive, need time alone, are mildly anti-social
- Thought is persistent and on-going: are philosophers
- Strong will-power, humanitarianism, care for ecology
- Your calcium genetics make you fine mental workers

- Either average or great achiever; some become homeless
- Appear passive, but are assertive (and may be aggressive)
- Poor memorization, but understand principles and natural law
- Desire fame and fortune; have executive and leadership abilities
- You seek friends who are non-combative, peaceful, philosophical
- Have an ability to endure: may be killed or maimed in battle, but are never mentally conquered!
- The males are sports minded in youth, but neither sex loves to exercise; males are more likely to be attached to relaxing
- Formal education is difficult: the mind is slow, but once the facts are obtained, you may produce greatness
- High combativeness is present: you appear peaceful, but actually are a sleeping storm; when aroused you may erupt with fury

▶ *Einstein dropped out of high school (he was probably bored silly); but his mind eventually penetrated the greatest secrets of time, matter and space! Obviously, you are not a clone of his brain, but you do have great potential which may, or may not, manifest as reality.*

———

Potential Challenges

▶ *Rocine: "You don't care what others think of you; you may be misjudged for your lazy attitude and behaviors, or for the way you stand, sit, or speak."*

You may have evolved from or not experienced these general faults, so do not dwell on them:

- Many have an intense sexual drive
- May be sarcastic or cruel in some instances
- Often are "wishy-washy" and "don't walk their talk"
- May be pushy, aggressive, unsympathetic, forceful, commanding
- To the casual observer you may seem to be a "nobody"; in actuality, you are brimming with undeveloped talents, skills, and potential!

▶ *If you relate to any of the above challenges, doing something to overcome them serves your evolution.*

———

Isogenic Stress Management

You have strong *mental* stress prevention providing a good ability not to internalize stress into your stomach, adrenals, and immune system. *Emotional* stress prevention is moderate, and any of the above challenges may need reprogramming help. *[If needing help managing these stresses, see my prior books.]*

Love

You are romantic, but have difficulty expressing deep feelings; you are often attracted to the *eldic, carbogenic, myogenic and nitropheric* types. The males, particularly, are highly-charged sexually.

Talents and Vocations

Abilities — *Arts, sciences, research, healing, management, religion*

Rocine reported, around 1900, that you are not artistic, but I have seen this to be untrue today.

▶ *I have known or observed you as: actors, artists, doctors, engineers, entrepreneurs, computer specialists, and middle management people.*

The type information cannot predict what or who you will become, but you are capable of bringing a creative excellence or brilliance to your life.

Inabilities — *'Mindless' work!*

You are unable to stay with boring or repetitive work; you need to stay in one place and do something interesting.

▶ *Rocine: "You are not tall, but are heavy set weighing heavily in proportion to your body size. You learn slowly and ponderously, but then apply your knowledge in an original manner. When you embrace working on a project, you reach a maximum intensity and can hardly stop because of your momentum."*

―――――

Isogenic Health Problems

When sick you commonly experience health problems or diseases in any of the following organs and tissues:

Skin — The male youth is usually inclined to pimples and boils.

Lymphatics — The lymph is your key health problem. You are inclined to lowered immune function from this cause (I knew two females of your type who had Hodgkin's disease).

Pancreas — Hypoglycemia is common (Rocine also found many diabetics in your type).

Infections — Chronic infections are common from Candida and Epstein-Barr virus, etc.

Liver — This organ is weak and inefficient: a semi-vegetarian diet without red meat helps your health.

Circulation — Your circulation is generally weak, although the heart is strong; you complain of cold feet.

Arthritis, Gout, Calcifications — You absorb calcium like a vacuum cleaner and end up with calcium deposits in joints and soft tissues (you need to limit your calcium intake).

▶ *I have seen acne or boils from lymphatic and immune problems to be a common finding in the male teenager; it may last for years. Exercise and diet is a healing key to lymph problems.*

Acid/Alkaline Factor

For your health and healing, your nervous system genetics require a specific ratio of acid to alkaline foods. You are born with **intermediate** dominance (between *para-sympathetic* and *sympathetic*), and need *balanced* acid and alkaline-ash food intake. (Ash refers to the minerals left in your body after metabolizing foods.) You may indulge in both food classes. Construct this approximate ratio of food selections:

50% Fruits, salads, vegetables
50% Proteins, carbohydrates

▶ *Approximate your food ratios. On any particular day, it does not matter if one meal is mostly alkaline and another mostly acid—just try to balance it out for the day! If you make a mistake, try again tomorrow. It is a subjective call that you make, as what you do over weeks and months makes the difference to your health.*

The Isogenic Spiritual Factor

Skip this paragraph if uninterested in a philosophical perspective on your type!

▶ *Rocine: "The soul chooses the body type."*

If as souls, we choose the brain and body type we spend a lifetime in, it could be to learn certain spiritual lessons related to perfecting ourselves, and our humanity (in God's eyes). If so, what lessons does this type bring for you. If this is your type, only you can really decide what those lessons are. You know what goes through your head, and how you behave towards others. You know your weaknesses and faults. You know things about yourself that Victor Rocine could never get his research subjects to admit to when he first wrote about types. So search your mind for the answer.

Each discrete type has life lessons, spiritual goals, etc., and your type challenges are often:

Humanity — Your focus on artistic or scientific work may outweigh your soul need for social and human communion.

Faith — Your faith is cerebral. You have a strong mental body, and you often conclude that believing in God is a stronger choice than not believing.

Sarcasm — You may have an unusual sense of humor. Some of you hurt others by saying or doing inconsiderate things.

Addiction — You may desire to experiment with hallucinogenic drugs: it is a spiritual challenge to deny yourself.

Overly-Intellectual and Lazy — Some of you would rather sit and think than do work; avoid doing nothing! Even if actively busy working, many males ache for peace and an armchair.

An Overly-Strong and Strident Voice — Your voice may be heard from a distance, and often annoyingly so. Accordingly, monitor your vocal tones —others will appreciate it!

———

An Isogenic Story…

James, age 39, 5'4, muscular, a little overweight, with a pock-marked face from childhood acne, drank excessive alcohol, and suffered from fatigue, headaches, and recurrent boils.

Examination showed a toxic liver and lymphatic system, for which he needed to stop pot and alcohol, or at least to cut his intake. His diet showed excessive calcium food intake from: Swiss and cheddar cheese, turnip greens, almonds, brewer's yeast, parsley, corn tortillas, dandelion greens, and Brazil nuts. He also ate excessively of salty junk foods: fast foods, canned, packaged, and frozen foods, soy sauce, meals, dill pickles, sauerkraut, and preserved meats.

James made these dietary changes, took the herbs, nutrients and food supplements indicated for his type to facilitate his healing. He entered an out-patient drug detox program with complete success.

Important Rocine Note

If unhealthy, eat 1-3 servings of these two food categories <u>daily</u>:

<u>Citric</u> *acid foods:*

Grapefruit, citron, limes, oranges, pomegranate, raspberries

<u>Formic</u> *acid foods:*

Avocado, cucumbers, mangos, pears, persimmons, pineapples
[If in good health be sure to eat these foods regularly.]

Isogenic Type
Mineral Needs

Apply this mineral data to the diet following the Fat type descriptions.

Excessive Foods:

- *Calcium*
- *Carbon (simple carbohydrates)*
- *Hydrogen*
- *Sodium, Chloride (salt, salted junk foods)*

Deficient Foods:

- *Magnesium*
- *Potassium*
- *Trace Minerals*
- *Sodium, Chloride (un-salted foods)*

These deficient minerals are common deficiencies in   your type, and predispose you to ill-health.
If ill, be sure to use these lists with your daily food intake.
If not ill, eat from the food lists 3-4 days weekly for health maintenance.
All food lists are in descending order of concentration and value to you; choose servings of foods in the upper half of each list first!
One serving is 1/2 cup.

Isogenic Excessive Foods -

Calcium is excessive in your tissues. It is highly concentrated in your bones, joints, muscles, nerves, heart, teeth, and gums. If you have an illness or disease in any of these tissues minimize calcium foods and supplements.

Carbon is excessive in your type, particularly simple carbohydrates, so minimize it. It is excessive in all people who become fat or obese, and is in every cell of your body as the basis of life. Generally:

Avoid <u>simple</u> *carbohydrates: white and brown sugars, high fructose corn syrup, honey, maple syrup, molasses, jellies, candy, ice cream, sodas.*
Eat <u>complex</u> *carbohydrates: yams, potatoes, squash, pumpkin, corn, lentils, peas, beans, green vegetables, grains.*

Hydrogen is excessive, particularly in females, contributing to obesity and water-logging of your tissues. Avoid iced drinks.

Sodium and chloride from salted junk foods is excessive in your tissues and contributes to aging, weight gain, and to negative mental and emotional states. To preserve your health and weight control you should avoid junk foods and fulfill your sodium needs from the food list (without using the salt-shaker).

Deficient Foods -

In illness or disease, it is important to correct these deficiencies.

Magnesium may be deficient in your type, and is particularly important for your brain, heart and digestive function.

Potassium is often deficient in your type. It is concentrated in and vital to the health of your muscles, heart, brain and all cells. If ill or diseased, potassium foods and supplements are an important healing factor.

Trace minerals easily become deficient in your type due to emotional stress or poor digestion and absorption.

Sodium and chloride from unsalted, non-junk foods is deficient.

[See the Appendix for descriptive notes and functions of minerals.]

———

<u>*Minimize*</u>

Excessive Foods

Calcium: *2-3 servings/<u>week</u>*

Swiss and cheddar cheese, turnip greens, dulse, greens (collard, turnip, dandelion, beet), almonds, parsley, Brazil nuts, watercress, celery, goat milk, tofu, dried figs, buttermilk, yogurt, wheat bran, whole milk, ripe olives.

Carbon, Hydrogen: *0-2 servings/week*

Carbohydrates, pumpkin, watermelon, celery, lettuce, alcohol, almonds, avocado, butter, most cereals, chocolate, cookies, pies, etc. (all white sugar foods), corn syrup, sweet fruits, cocoa, coconuts, cheeses, corn, currant, cream, dates, egg yolk, honey, legumes, margarine, nuts.

Sodium, Chloride (salted, junk):
   0-1 servings/week

Salt, all fast foods, packaged foods, canned and frozen foods, soy sauce, all preserved meats (cured, smoked, canned and luncheon meats), sauces (barbecue, catsup, etc.), dill pickles, sauerkraut, bouillon cubes, peanut butter, potato chips, etc., salted nuts, crackers, canned or packaged soups, processed cheeses.

<u>Eat</u>

Deficient Foods

Magnesium, Potassium: *1-2 servings/day*

Blackstrap molasses, buckwheat, legumes, nuts, dulse, filberts, millet and whole grains, asparagus (cooked), beet greens, spinach, pumpkin seeds, figs, brown rice, Swiss chard, apricots (dried), cantaloupe, potato, pinto beans, bananas, kidney beans, dates, shrimp.

Trace Minerals: *1-2 servings/day*

Kelp, clams, crabs, raw cabbage, raw cauliflower, cod liver oil, goat's cheese and milk, raw garlic, sprouts, mussels, oysters, scallops, sorrel, blackberries, lean meats, liver, deep-green leafy vegetables, sprouts, egg yolk, asparagus.

Sodium, Chloride (unsalted, non-junk): *1-2 servings/day*

Scallops, lobster, gizzard, celery and juice, Swiss chard, milk, kelp, olives, lobster, beets and greens, egg whites, cod, salt water fish, lamb, pistachio (unsalted), turkey, okra, turnips (not greens), carrots, strawberry.

Note - *Drink warm or hot citrus juices (preferred over water).*

Isogenic Nutritional Supplements

- **Multi-Vitamins** — *[Take all supplements with food.]*— *2 capsules/day*

- **Potassium** — *99 mg/day*

- **Magnesium** *– 100 mg/day*

- **Do not take Calcium or Multi-Minerals —**

  Your body has excessive calcium/minerals.. (Exception: high stress, menopause, on estrogen, osteoporotic)

- **Herbs** —

  Brain detox – Valerian Root or Gotu Kola
  Organ detox – Chickweed or Milk Thistle
  (Take one capsule, twice daily for one month; then one, three times weekly.)

- **Evening Primrose or Flaxseed Oil** *— Take one soft-gel/day with food*

- **Other** —

  Chlorophyll, blue-green algae, green magma, spirulina, alfalfa, or other source.

  (Take as directed; or get liquid trace minerals, and take once daily.)

Important Isogenic Health Concerns

Your nervous system genetics require the *Fat* type Food Guide for health; while young, any carnivorous cravings are healthy for you, but after about age 40, you need a partial vegetarian diet with 2-3 flesh days each week.

ISOGENIC FOOD GUIDE

Aim for –

50% Proteins, complex carbohydrates
50% Fruits, salads, vegetables
and
50% Raw food diet
50% Cooked foods

Lose the salt shaker.
Exercise is essential for your health.
Take the recommended supplements.

▶ *Rocine: "You thrive on citrus fruit and drinks, strawberries, cooked foods, coarse whole grain breads and honey. You need to <u>avoid</u> fats, salt, white sugar foods, carbohydrates, alcohol, and drugs."*

Isogenic Weight Loss

Your body absorbs excessive fat from an early age, and you have great difficulty in losing it. Give yourself permission to exercise! It is essential for your fat burning. You will make good progress with the above *Food Guide* and by following these instructions:

- *Gluten* is often an allergic factor
- *Avoid* simple carbohydrates, junk sodium foods (see list)
- *Avoid* all foods that can be juiced (see list)
- *Protein* drink in citrus juice daily, about 25-30 grams
- *Eat* your body type deficient mineral foods daily
- *Follow* your *Isogenic Guide (as above)*
- *Exercise*: your body type requires <u>intense</u> daily exercise for health and for weight loss
- *Simple sugars*: stop all white table sugar and high-fructose corn syrup and drinks containing these sugars
- *Instead of diet pills,* you need glucomanin supplements that swell and take up space in the stomach thus preventing over-eating
- *If hypoglycemic* (low blood sugar, fatigue, depression, etc.), which stops fat loss and usually initiates more fat production, it is vital to deal with this problem: take *pantothenic acid,* 500 mg/twice daily with

food (see my earlier books to resolve this problem)

- *Calories:* As with any dietary approach, calories in, must be *less than* calories out! Most markets sell a calorie booklet; make notes of your daily intake, and in most instances keep it under about 1500-1800 calories/day

―――

Fat Types
General Food Guide

*(An Intermediate Guide between
Carnivores and Vegetarians)*

Important Note

———

The Food Guide addresses the <u>*Acid-Alkaline*</u> aspect of your food intake, along with the <u>*Type Mineral*</u> factor presented throughout this book. It does <u>*not*</u> necessarily address calories or other dietary factors that may be pertinent to your personal health needs whether medical or appropriate for some other dietary need. So use your common sense and just include the factors described here with whatever healthy dietary choices you usually make.

For other nutrient information, consult with nutritional books or with holistic nutritional doctors. In this regard, I particularly recommend the advice of Andrew Weil, M.D.

———

Fat Types
General Food Guide

*This chapter presents an <u>Intermediate</u> Food Guide,
balanced between the Muscle types (carnivores) and the Thin
types (vegetarians). Superimpose the individual type mineral
and other information from your type chapter into this Food
Guide (which is not for the pargenic type.)*

Meat/Flesh Intake

Generally, animal protein is acceptable and
needed in your diet: red meat should be
limited to once weekly or less, while lamb and
fish or poultry are excellent in moderation. If
this diet is similar to what you are already eating,
but you have health problems because of a
history of excess acid-ash food intake being so
common, then:

- Decrease your carbohydrate and
  protein intake by about one-third
- Increase your fruit, salad and vegetable
  intake by about one-third
- Consult with a holistic doctor,
  preferably one versed in nutritional and
  emotional evaluation

Over-Acid or Over-Alkaline?

Just as a log of wood burned in your fireplace leaves a mineral-ash, food ash refers to the minerals remaining after metabolizing foods in your tissues:

- Fruits and vegetables **alkalinize** tissues
- Proteins and carbohydrates **acidify** tissues

You are usually over-acid due to:

- Accumulated metabolic waste-acids
- Deficient fruit, salad and vegetable intake
- Excessive protein and carbohydrate intake

You need to estimate the ratio of foods you are eating: generally, eat the following *approximate* ratio of foods for your health:

50% *Alkaline-ash* foods (fruits, salads, vegetables)
50% *Acid-ash* foods (complex carbohydrates like starches, grains, cereals, breads, flour products; and proteins)

Approximate your food ratios. On any particular day it does not matter if one meal is mostly alkaline, and another is acid—just try to balance it out for the day! If you make a mistake, forget it and try again tomorrow. It is a subjective call that you make. It is what you do over weeks and months that makes the difference to your health—not on any few days.

The net result is that the Fat types require the plan presented in this chapter for health restoration.

[The following chart shows the fat types, their acid-alkaline reactions, and the percentage of raw foods needed for their healing.]

Fat Types

Acid/Alkaline Genetics Dietary-Ash and Raw Food Needs

This chart shows the Rocine types, their acid or alkaline food needs, and the percentage of raw foods needed for your health and healing.

BODY TYPE	ACID/ALKALINE GENETICS	% DIET ASH	% RAW FOODS
Barotic	*Intermediate*	*50:50*	*50*
Carboferic	*Intermediate*	*50:50*	*50*
Hydripheric	*Intermediate*	*50:50*	*30*
Isogenic	*Intermediate*	*50:50*	*30*
Lipopheric	*Intermediate*	*50:50*	*50*
Oxypheric	*Intermediate*	*50:50*	*50*
Pargenic	*Acid*	*70% alkaline*	*30*

Note that the above percentages will vary depending on aging and the health of individual types.

Notes

- Never eat foods you are allergic to, no matter what I recommend here; if you suspect allergy to a suggested food, eliminate it.
- Minimize your white sugar and alcohol intake.
- Eat the right foods most of the time and the diet will help you; you do not have to live out of a health food store (although such foods are healthier).
- All food lists are in descending order of concentration and value to you as a mineral source; whenever possible, choose foods in the upper half of each list first! One serving is ½ cup.
- If desired, you may interchange lunches for dinners.
- Avoid all junk foods, white sugar, foods with added sugar, and high fructose corn syrup

———

General Food Guide
Breakfast

EGGS (1-2) with lettuce, tomato, whole grain toast — 1-3 times/week; or

FRUIT SALAD, fresh with citrus fruit and a protein source (low-sugar yogurt, kefir, milk, cottage cheese, cheese, seeds or nuts) — 2-4 times/week; or

COOKED CEREALS, fruit, seeds, whole grain, and nuts — 2-5 times/week; or

OTHER — 0-1 times/week

Eat unlimited fruit, salads, vegetables, with seeds/nuts for snacks. Wheat is a common allergy: avoid white and wheat breads; eat rye, sour dough, or oat breads instead

* * *

DAILY LIQUIDS

Pure water — as desired (except Hydripheric type)
Fruit and vegetable juices — 0-2 cups
Coffee, caffeine teas — 0-2 cups

[Include selections from your type mineral needs with each meal.]

Lunch

SALADS, mixed green, and 2-4 oz., of protein (fish, poultry, egg, cheese, tofu, seeds or nuts, etc.) [Dressings: use canola or olive oil* and vinegar; or low-fat/calorie dressing] — 2-4 times/week; or

VEGETABLES (steamed) with salad, and yogurt, or cottage cheese (or other breakfast proteins) — 1-2 times/week; or

FRUIT SALAD (see breakfast) — 0-1 times/week

SANDWICH, whole grains with a non-flesh protein (egg, tofu, cheese, etc.) —1-3 times/week; or

POULTRY, FISH, 3-4 oz., with a mixed green salad and/or steamed vegetables (or as a sandwich) —1-2 times/week; or

OTHER — 0-1 times/week

* Other oils less ideal; soybean is common allergen; minimize commercial dressings

[Include selections from your type mineral needs with each meal.]

Dinner

LEAN POULTRY OR FISH (4-6 oz.)
— 2-4 times/week

PASTA, PROTEIN (as above)
—1-3 times/week

VEGETARIAN MEAL, including legumes, tofu,
cheese, cottage cheese, seeds or nuts, egg, etc.
—2-4 times/week

LEAN BEEF (4-6 oz.) — 0-2 times/month

OTHER — 0-2 times/week

Take all of the above with: mixed green salad,
dressing (as before), and/or vegetables (steamed are
best).

DESSERTS

Fruits, fresh — as desired
Low-sugar, healthy desserts — 0-3 times/week

If you have blood fat problems, cholesterol or
triglycerides, eliminate all beef from your diet, and
see my earlier books.

Eat fruit, unlimited salads and vegetables with
seeds/nuts, low-sugar yogurt for snacks.

[Include selections from your type mineral
needs with each meal.]

Fat Types Notes

Do not eat flesh everyday: have it on alternate days only. For munchies, have low calorie items like celery and other vegetables, along with yogurt and cottage cheese, etc. Some of you abuse your beef and red meat intake, perhaps several times weekly—this is a false craving; use your will to combat it if you want to be healthier!

Steamed Vegetables —Minerals are lost in the boiling of vegetables; best is steaming or wok cooking.

Minimize Foods — Only eat them 0-1 times/week! Be sure to eat the recommended foods to help your healing;

Food Combinations —Eating proteins at the same meal with starches often results in indigestion, gas or constipation (along with low blood sugar and making fat). Watch how this inharmonious food combination may be affecting you.

Minimize —

- All fatty foods
- Milk and dairy foods (unless otherwise noted)
- Commercial, sugared, and fatty salad dressings
- Beef, sugar, wines, alcohol, coffee, white sugar, red meats, and processed meats

Vegetarian Proteins — If you choose to be vegetarian, it will help your health after middle-age; because you have semi-carnivorous genes be sure to take a protein supplement of 20-30 grams/day (e.g., soy or egg-white powder in juice).

Healthy Weight — Invariably you hold excessive weight, and in addition to body type factors there may be a medical problem behind your fat storage. By eating according to your body type, you slowly and naturally lose excess weight! Accumulating evidence indicts high-fructose corn syrup as a major cause of increased weight and obesity. Avoid it!

You have a sluggish fat-burning metabolism, and may have an under-active adrenal, thyroid, or pituitary gland resulting in hypoglycemia, and in this instance may need the services of a holistic doctor *(see Appendix* and my earlier books).

———

In Conclusion

I hope you have enjoyed reading this book. You should now know your body type and have learned some valuable information about how to be a healthier you! Do not forget the advice on page 10, along with my previous books on healing yourself.

If you desire further help or information with your body type or health from a holistic viewpoint, email me from page one of my web page: Dr.Stenbeck.net

Good health and good luck!

———

Appendix

Brief Extracts from
The 22 Unique Body Types

Appendix A

Types
(Brief extract)

Type comes from 'typus' meaning an image or impression, the study of types being called typology.

▶ *Rocine: "A combination of mental and structural features is consistently found in people of the same type."*

Rocine wrote that all types are a mixture of positive and negative qualities. He based his work on the biochemical individuality of our *mineral* absorption and utilization. Of course, all minerals are absorbed, but he postulated that different types of people *selectively* absorb certain minerals, to a greater or lesser extent, requiring specific mineral foods for their enhanced health and healing.

▶ *The type information cannot predict what or who you will become, or how successful or not, but your type is capable of bringing a creative excellence to whatever you do in life. If your type has negative qualities that you disagree with, remember that they are only tendencies and may or may not manifest in you.*

This book enlarges on Rocine's premise (early 1900's), integrated with the later research of Herbert Sheldon, M.D., Ph.D., at Harvard University (1930's), along with my fifty years of observations and experience with this subject.

Comparing your shared physical (and sometimes psychological) descriptions with the Celebrity Lists further assists the identification of your type. It is not that you will look exactly like, or be a twin to, any particular celebrity. Look closely at a celebrity's features: face, profile, height, weight, head, etc. If you know something about their talents, beliefs, success and failure spheres, health and weight challenges, attitudes and behaviors, etc., then you get clues as to what your type may be.

———

Understanding Types and Sub-Types

Each of us has a clearly discernible dominant type. Visualize the celebrity examples from movies, politics, sports, the arts and public life, and try to identify with their physical features. Look for similar features, remembering that you will not recognize all attributes in yourself. You are not looking for your twin!

The sub-type issue is the main reason people of the same major type can look so different. Remember that a type description does not characterize you exactly, but depicts your individual variant of a type.

▶ *The type questionnaire pinpoints the major features of that type: if the celebrity examples are unhelpful, you may be an unusual variant (in which case ignore the celebrity issue and give yourself 7 points on Question 1).*

———

Minerals

Minerals are essential life nutrients that accelerate enzyme and chemical reactions and provide a basis for your body typing. Although found in all tissues, different minerals tend to be concentrated in certain organs, their presence or absence contributing to the healing of such tissues; e.g., zinc accelerates prostate healing; calcium and manganese promote bone, joint and connective tissue healing.

Specific foods nurture each type, some people needing meats for their health others needing a vegetarian diet. A high potassium diet nurtures one person, while another needs high sulfur, calcium, zinc, or another mineral.

Mineral Digestion and Absorption

Compared to vitamins, minerals are *difficult* to digest, absorb, and utilize. In people with strong digestive systems, this aspect may not be important. The following factors should be in place for optimal mineral metabolism:

1. Stomach Hydrochloric Acid Production
2. Parathyroid Hormone Balance
3. Organ Toxic Metal and Chemical Removal
   [See details in The 22 Unique Body Types.]

————

Total Body Healing

Note that from a holistic healing perspective, in addition to minerals and type information, the following healing factors are necessary:

> *Nutrient Balance*
> *Mental Balance*
> *Emotional Balance*
> *Spiritual Balance*
> *Detoxifying Integrity*

The above factors are all important to your total healing especially if you are interested in self-healing (see my earlier books).

————

Appendix B

Researchers
(Brief extract)

The predominant workers in this area of human individuality from around 1880's to the 1960's are Herbert Sheldon, M.D., Ph.D., Roger Williams, Ph.D., and Victor Rocine, D.Sc.

Much information on Sheldon's research exists on-line and in medical psychology libraries; for interested readers there are other lines of research published in the last century. This present book is primarily about Rocine's body types.

Herbert Sheldon M.D., Ph.D.

In contrast to Rocine, Sheldon at Harvard University in the 1930's was trained in the scientific method and did painstaking research and publishing on human individuality. In comparing his findings with Rocine's work, a direct putative correlation is visible.

Roger J. Williams, Ph.D.

Another significant researcher in human individuality is the renowned scientist and biochemist, Roger J. Williams. He demonstrated that different people have varying levels of nutrients, enzymes, and other metabolic chemicals in their bloodstreams.

▶ *Williams's research firmly expands on the premise of individual nutritional needs in human beings. If interested in his research, I highly recommend his book <u>Biochemial Individuality</u>.*

Victor Rocine, D.Sc.

Note that when a negative feature is indicated, say neurotic tendencies, all members of the type are <u>not</u> that way; it is a type tendency reported by Rocine.

Rocine studied type-related diseases finding links between mineral and dietary factors with individual types and their diseases. In each body type, one or more dominant minerals are preferentially absorbed and utilized over other minerals.

He recognized discrete body types from their physical appearance finding genetically based mineral dominance to be the determining feature. He also correlated their physical features with psychological characteristics.

———

Appendix C
Genetics, Types, and Diet
(Brief extract)

This section deals with how nervous system genetics helps determine your eating choices for health: you are either born to be a predominant meat eater, a partial or complete vegetarian, or something between the two. The genetic factor determining this dietary aspect is the *sympathetic and parasympathetic* components of your central nervous system. This represents a basic factor in eating for health.

This chapter helps you understand your dietary inheritance, although instinctively, you may already have arrived there!

- If born **sympathetic** dominant you are *genetically acid*, desiring a predominantly *vegetarian* diet for your health (about 70% fruit, salad, vegetables to 30% proteins and carbohydrates).

- If born **parasympathetic** dominant you are *genetically alkaline*, desiring a predominantly *carnivorous* diet for your health (about 70% proteins, carbohydrates to 30% fruits, salads, vegetables). Few of you ever choose to become vegetarian because of the difficulty in satisfying your protein needs without meats.

- If born ***intermediate*** dominant you
  may eat food groups with little concern
  for the acid/alkaline factor. However,
  after age 40, you need a semi-vegetarian
  diet for healthy eating.

———

Chart of Relative Nervous System Dominance

In the following Chart, if you relate to many
of the symptoms on one side you probably
have that nervous system dominance; relating
to both sides indicates *Intermediate* dominance.

If Vegetarian (Over-acid) --
> *Eat 70% fruits, salads, vegetables*
> *And 30% proteins, carbohydrates*

If Carnivore (Over-alkaline) --
> *Eat 70% proteins, carbohydrates*
> *And 30% fruits, salads, vegetables*

If Intermediate --
> *Eat 50:50 of acid and alkaline-ash foods*

Make an *approximate* estimate of your daily
acid and alkaline food intake (such ratios varying
from type to type).

———

Symptoms of Relative Genetic Dominance

Vegetarians (Over-acid)	Carnivores (Over-alkaline)
Sympathetic Dominance	*Parasympathetic Dominance*
little or no flesh desire	desire flesh
easily constipated	rarely constipated
slow digestion	fast digestion
easily dehydrated	not dehydrated
strong thirst	low thirst
pale face	flushed face
high pulse after food	slow pulse after food
easy gag reflex	slow gag reflex
cool dry skin	moist warm skin
nervous stomach	calm stomach
little eyelid blinking	much blinking
nervous tendency	mostly calm
slower healing	faster healing
low oxygen-uptake	good oxygen-uptake
easily breathless	seldom breathless
insomnia common	sleep easier
few muscle cramps	some night cramps
calcium deposits rare	get calcium deposits

Appendix D

Help Identifying your Body Type with Dr. Stenbeck

If you desire help in identifying your body type, follow these instructions, and answer the questionnaire. For further information and fees, send me an email from page one of the website:

DrStenbeck.net

First name: _____

Country of birth: _____

Upload photos and send to the above website:

- Head and shoulders: front and side views

- Full body: front and side views

- Also 1-2 teenage views

- If possible, casual photos of mother, father, siblings

MY TYPE CLASS MAY BE: _____

   (Thin, Muscle, or Fat)

AGE   -   _____

HEIGHT   -   _____ feet/inches

MY WEIGHT -   _____ pounds

   Heaviest at age: _____

- Lightest as adult: _____

- Estimate age 15: _____

VISION - Excellent Average   Poor:

HAIR -   Natural color: _____   -

- Thin/thick? _____

- balding? _____

SKIN - Quality: _____

- History of acne, boils, other:

_____

_____

TEETH   - Strong   Weak   Dentures

- Cavity history: Many   Moderate   Few

MUSCLES - Strong   Average   Weak

Sports played _____

JOINTS   - Strong   Average   Weak

HEALTH - Childhood diseases?

_____

_____

- Adult diseases?

_____

AVERAGE DIET

- Beef   _____ (times/week)

 - Poultry   _____ (times/week)

 - Fish   _____ (times/week)

 - Eggs   _____ (times/week)

 - Water   _____ (glasses/day):

 - Vegetarian? Vegan?   _____

 - Other?   _____

- Did your childhood diet differ? _____

The above will help me know who you are! I will send you a follow-up questionnaire for further help in identifying your body type.

Appendix E

On-line Health Consultation
with Dr. Stenbeck

For further information, or to comment on this book, or to receive a response on any health issue from a holistic viewpoint, send an email inquiry from page one of my website:

DrStenbeck.net

Following that, I will suggest further healing needs, which we may pursue with an on-line consult.

———

Appendix F

Notes

See my book *The 22 Unique Body Types*, available at the usual online source, for further information and details on all of the 22 Types. The Appendix in that book has further information about:

Mineral Functions and Food Sources

Further Reading

———